UNMASKING PARKINSON'S DISEASE

Navigating the Complexities of a Neurological Disorder, Understanding, Coping, and Thriving with the Neurodegenerative Disease

Anita Hulsey

Table Of Contents

INTRODUCTION

In the bustling tapestry of life, Simon emerges as a central figure, a protagonist whose narrative is both inspiring and challenging. Parkinson's Disease, a formidable adversary, casts its shadow over his path, introducing uncertainty and complexity where once there was only routine and familiarity. Yet, in the face of this daunting diagnosis, Simon stands resolute, a beacon of strength and resilience in a sea of uncertainty.

As he embarks on his journey to unmask the intricacies of Parkinson's Disease, Simon discovers a profound truth: that the key to combating this condition lies not only in medical interventions but also in the transformative power of nutrition. Thus, with a heart full of determination and a mind brimming with curiosity, he sets out to explore the boundless realm of culinary possibilities, seeking solace and strength in the nurturing embrace of wholesome foods.

Breakfast, the herald of a new day, becomes a canvas upon which Simon paints his first strokes of defiance against the encroaching shadows of Parkinson's. From vibrant smoothies bursting with antioxidants to hearty oatmeal infused with the sweetness of berries, each morning meal is a testament to Simon's unwavering commitment to his well-being.

As the sun reaches its zenith, Simon's journey continues through the realm of lunch, where salads teeming with grilled salmon and bowls brimming with quinoa and vibrant vegetables offer sustenance and vitality in equal measure. Here, amidst the hustle and bustle of midday, Simon finds a moment of respite, a chance to refuel both body and soul in preparation for the challenges that lie ahead.

And as twilight descends, casting a gentle glow over the horizon, Simon's culinary odyssey reaches its crescendo with dinner. Baked chicken nestled alongside sweet potatoes, fragrant lentil soup adorned with tender kale, and succulent cod paired with roasted vegetables—all serve as testaments to the richness and diversity of flavors that can nourish not just the body, but also the spirit.

In the quiet moments between meals, Simon discovers the power of snacks—small yet potent morsels that offer sustenance and comfort in times of need. Greek yogurt with almonds, crisp carrot sticks dipped in creamy hummus, apple slices adorned with velvety peanut butter, and trail mix bursting with dried fruits and nuts—all stand as reminders of the abundance of nourishment that surrounds him.

Through these culinary creations, Simon weaves a tapestry of healing and hope, inviting others to join him on this transformative journey towards unmasking Parkinson's Disease. In each recipe, in each shared moment of vulnerability and triumph, Simon's story resonates—a testament to the indomitable human spirit and the power of nourishment, both physical and emotional, in the face of adversity. Together, let us walk alongside Simon as he navigates the complexities of Parkinson's, one meal at a time, one shared experience at a time, forging a path towards wellness, understanding, and ultimately, triumph.

CHAPTER ONE

Breakfast Recipes for Parkinson's Patients

-Energizing Smoothie

Recipe 1:

Berry Blast Energizing Smoothie

Nutritional Information:
- Calories: 200
- Protein: 5g
- Carbohydrates: 35g
- Fat: 3g

Cooking Time: 5 minutes
Serving Size: 1

Ingredients:
- 1 cup mixed berries (strawberries, blueberries, raspberries)
- 1 ripe banana
- 1/2 cup Greek yogurt
- 1 tablespoon honey
- 1/2 cup almond milk
- Ice cubes

Instructions:
1. Add all ingredients into a blender.
2. Blend until smooth and creamy.
3. Pour into a glass and enjoy immediately.

Recipe 2:

Green Power Energizing Smoothie

Nutritional Information:
- Calories: 180
- Protein: 8g
- Carbohydrates: 30g
- Fat: 4g

Cooking Time: 5 minutes
Serving Size: 1

Ingredients:
- 1 cup spinach
- 1/2 cucumber
- 1/2 avocado
- 1/2 lime, juiced
- 1 tablespoon chia seeds
- 1 cup coconut water
- Ice cubes

Instructions:
1. Combine all ingredients in a blender.
2. Blend until smooth and creamy.
3. Serve in a glass and enjoy the freshness.

 Recipe 3:

Tropical Sunshine Energizing Smoothie

Nutritional Information:
- Calories: 220

- Protein: 4g
- Carbohydrates: 45g
- Fat: 2g

Cooking Time: 5 minutes
Serving Size: 1

Ingredients:
- 1/2 cup pineapple chunks
- 1/2 cup mango chunks
- 1/2 banana
- 1/2 cup orange juice
- 1/4 cup coconut milk
- Ice cubes

Instructions:
1. Put all ingredients in a blender.
2. Blend until smooth and creamy.
3. Pour into a glass and enjoy the tropical flavors.

Recipe 4:

Nutty Protein Energizing Smoothie

Nutritional Information:
- Calories: 250
- Protein: 12g
- Carbohydrates: 30g
- Fat: 8g

Cooking Time: 5 minutes
Serving Size:1

Ingredients:
- 1 banana
- 2 tablespoons peanut butter
- 1 tablespoon cocoa powder
- 1/2 cup oats
- 1 cup milk of choice
- Ice cubes

Instructions:
1. Combine all ingredients in a blender.
2. Blend until smooth and creamy.
3. Pour into a glass and enjoy the nutty goodness.

Oatmeal with Berries

Recipe 1:

 Blueberry Oatmeal Delight

Nutritional Information:
- Calories: 300
- Protein: 10g
- Carbohydrates: 50g
- Fat: 5g

Cooking Time: 10 minutes
Serving Size: 1

Ingredients:
- 1/2 cup rolled oats
- 1 cup water
- 1/2 cup fresh blueberries
- 1 tablespoon honey
- 1 tablespoon chopped nuts (e.g., almonds or walnuts)
- Pinch of cinnamon

Instructions:

1. In a small saucepan, bring water to a boil.
2. Add oats and reduce heat to low. Cook for 5 minutes, stirring occasionally.
3. Stir in blueberries and continue cooking for another 2-3 minutes until the oats are creamy.
4. Remove from heat and stir in honey.
5. Transfer oatmeal to a bowl, top with chopped nuts and a sprinkle of cinnamon.
6. Enjoy your nutritious and delicious blueberry oatmeal!

Recipe 2:

 Strawberry Banana Oatmeal Bowl

Nutritional Information:
- Calories: 320
- Protein: 8g
- Carbohydrates: 55g
- Fat: 6g

Cooking Time: 10 minutes

Serving Size: 1

Ingredients:
- 1/2 cup rolled oats
- 1 cup milk of choice
- 1/2 banana, sliced
- 1/2 cup sliced strawberries
- 1 tablespoon maple syrup
- 1 tablespoon flax seeds

Instructions:
1. In a saucepan, combine oats and milk. Bring to a simmer over medium heat.
2. Cook for about 5-7 minutes or until the oats are creamy, stirring occasionally.
3. Add sliced banana and continue cooking for another 1-2 minutes.
4. Remove from heat and transfer to a bowl.
5. Top with sliced strawberries, drizzle with maple syrup, and sprinkle flax seeds on top.
6. Enjoy your delicious and nutritious strawberry banana oatmeal bowl!

Recipe 3:

Raspberry Almond Oatmeal

Nutritional Information:
- Calories: 280
- Protein: 7g
- Carbohydrates: 45g
- Fat: 8g

Cooking Time: 10 minutes
Serving Size: 1

Ingredients:
- 1/2 cup rolled oats
- 1 cup almond milk
- 1/2 cup fresh raspberries
- 1 tablespoon almond butter
- 1 tablespoon honey
- Sliced almonds for garnish

Instructions:
1. In a saucepan, combine oats and almond milk. Bring to a gentle boil.

2. Reduce heat and simmer for 5-7 minutes, stirring occasionally.

3. Add fresh raspberries and almond butter, stirring until well combined.

4. Cook for another 1-2 minutes until the raspberries soften.

5. Remove from heat, stir in honey, and transfer to a bowl.

6. Top with sliced almonds for added crunch and enjoy your raspberry almond oatmeal!

Recipe 4:

Mixed Berry Chia Oatmeal

Nutritional Information:
- Calories: 330
- Protein: 9g
- Carbohydrates: 55g
- Fat: 7g

Cooking Time: 10 minutes
Serving Size: 1

Ingredients:
- 1/2 cup rolled oats
- 1 cup water
- 1/2 cup mixed berries (strawberries, blueberries, raspberries)
- 1 tablespoon chia seeds
- 1 tablespoon agave syrup
- Splash of milk (optional)

Instructions:
1. In a saucepan, combine oats and water. Bring to a boil, then reduce heat and simmer for 5-7 minutes.
2. Add mixed berries and chia seeds, stirring well.
3. Cook for another 2-3 minutes until the berries are softened.
4. Remove from heat, stir in agave syrup.
5. If desired, add a splash of milk for creaminess.
6. Transfer to a bowl and enjoy your mixed berry chia oatmeal, packed with goodness!

- Scrambled Eggs with Spinach

Recipe 1:

Classic Scrambled Eggs with Spinach

Nutritional Information:
- Calories: 250
- Protein: 15g
- Carbohydrates: 4g
- Fat: 18g

Cooking Time: 10 minutes
Serving Size: 1

Ingredients:
- 2 eggs
- 1 cup fresh spinach, chopped
- 1 tablespoon butter
- Salt and pepper to taste
- Optional: Shredded cheese for topping

Instructions:

1. In a bowl, whisk the eggs until well beaten. Season with salt and pepper.
2. Heat butter in a non-stick skillet over medium heat.
3. Add the chopped spinach to the skillet and sauté until wilted.
4. Pour in the beaten eggs and gently stir with a spatula as they begin to set.
5. Continue cooking and stirring until the eggs are cooked to your desired consistency.
6. Transfer to a plate, sprinkle with shredded cheese if desired, and serve hot.
7. Enjoy your classic scrambled eggs with spinach!

 Recipe 2:

Spinach and Feta Scrambled Eggs

Nutritional Information:
- Calories: 280
- Protein: 17g

- Carbohydrates: 5g
- Fat: 20g

Cooking Time: 15 minutes
Serving Size: 1

Ingredients:
- 2 eggs
- 1 cup fresh spinach, chopped
- 2 tablespoons crumbled feta cheese
- 1 tablespoon olive oil
- Salt and pepper to taste

Instructions:
1. In a bowl, whisk the eggs and season with salt and pepper.
2. Heat olive oil in a skillet over medium heat.
3. Add the chopped spinach and sauté until wilted.
4. Pour in the beaten eggs and cook, stirring gently until the eggs are almost set.

5. Sprinkle the crumbled feta cheese over the eggs and continue cooking for another minute.
6. Remove from heat, transfer to a plate, and serve hot.
7. Enjoy your flavorful spinach and feta scrambled eggs!

Recipe 3:

Creamy Spinach Scrambled Eggs

Nutritional Information:
- Calories: 270
- Protein: 16g
- Carbohydrates: 6g
- Fat: 19g

Cooking Time: 12 minutes
Serving Size: 1

Ingredients:
- 2 eggs
- 1/2 cup fresh spinach, chopped
- 2 tablespoons cream cheese

- 1 tablespoon butter
- Salt and pepper to taste

Instructions:
1. In a bowl, whisk the eggs and season with salt and pepper.
2. Heat butter in a skillet over medium heat.
3. Add the chopped spinach and sauté until wilted.
4. Pour in the beaten eggs and cook, stirring gently.
5. When the eggs are almost set, add the cream cheese and continue cooking until creamy.
6. Remove from heat, transfer to a plate, and serve hot.
7. Enjoy your rich and creamy spinach scrambled eggs!

Recipe 4:

Mushroom Spinach Scrambled Eggs

Nutritional Information:

- Calories: 290
- Protein: 18g
- Carbohydrates: 7g
- Fat: 21g

Cooking Time: 15 minutes
Serving Size: 1

Ingredients:
- 2 eggs
- 1 cup fresh spinach, chopped
- 1/2 cup mushrooms, sliced
- 1 tablespoon butter
- Salt and pepper to taste

Instructions:
1. In a bowl, whisk the eggs and season with salt and pepper.
2. Heat butter in a skillet over medium heat.
3. Add the sliced mushrooms and sauté until golden brown.
4. Add the chopped spinach and cook until wilted.

5. Pour in the beaten eggs and cook, stirring gently.
6. Cook until the eggs are set and everything is well combined.
7. Transfer to a plate, season with more salt and pepper if needed, and serve hot.
8. Enjoy your savory mushroom and spinach scrambled eggs!

- Banana Nut Chia Pudding

Recipe 1:

Classic Banana Nut Chia Pudding

Nutritional Information:
- Calories: 280
- Protein: 8g
- Carbohydrates: 35g
- Fat: 12g

Cooking Time: 5 minutes (plus chilling time)
Serving Size: 1

Ingredients:
- 1 ripe banana, mashed
- 2 tablespoons chia seeds
- 1/2 cup almond milk
- 1 tablespoon chopped nuts (e.g., walnuts, almonds)
- 1 tablespoon honey or maple syrup
- Dash of cinnamon

Instructions:
1. In a bowl, mix the mashed banana, chia seeds, almond milk, and honey.
2. Stir well to combine all ingredients.
3. Let the mixture sit for 5 minutes, then stir again to prevent clumping.
4. Cover and refrigerate for at least 2 hours or overnight.
5. Before serving, sprinkle with chopped nuts and a dash of cinnamon.
6. Enjoy your classic banana nut chia pudding!

Recipe 2:

Chocolate Banana Nut Chia Pudding

Nutritional Information:
- Calories: 320
- Protein: 9g
- Carbohydrates: 40g
- Fat: 15g

Cooking Time: 5 minutes (plus chilling time)
Serving Size: 1

Ingredients:
- 1 ripe banana, mashed
- 2 tablespoons chia seeds
- 1/2 cup coconut milk
- 1 tablespoon cocoa powder
- 1 tablespoon chopped nuts (e.g., pecans, hazelnuts)
- 1 tablespoon honey or agave syrup

Instructions:
1. In a bowl, mix the mashed banana, chia seeds, coconut milk, cocoa powder, and honey.

2. Stir well to combine all ingredients.
3. Let the mixture sit for 5 minutes, then stir again.
4. Cover and refrigerate for at least 2 hours or overnight.
5. Before serving, sprinkle with chopped nuts for extra crunch.
6. Indulge in the rich flavors of chocolate banana nut chia pudding!

Recipe 3:

Vanilla Banana Nut Chia Pudding Parfait

Nutritional Information:
- Calories: 300
- Protein: 8g
- Carbohydrates: 38g
- Fat: 14g

Cooking Time: 5 minutes (plus chilling time)
Serving Size: 1

Ingredients:
- 1 ripe banana, mashed
- 2 tablespoons chia seeds
- 1/2 cup vanilla almond milk
- 1 tablespoon chopped mixed nuts
- 1 tablespoon honey or maple syrup
- Granola (optional)

Instructions:
1. In a bowl, mix the mashed banana, chia seeds, vanilla almond milk, and honey.
2. Stir well to combine all ingredients.
3. Let the mixture sit for 5 minutes, then stir again.
4. Cover and refrigerate for at least 2 hours or overnight.
5. Before serving, layer the chia pudding with chopped nuts and granola in a glass.
6. Enjoy the delightful layers of vanilla banana nut chia pudding parfait!

Recipe 4:

Coconut Banana Nut Chia Pudding

Nutritional Information:
- Calories: 290
- Protein: 7g
- Carbohydrates: 36g
- Fat: 16g

Cooking Time: 5 minutes (plus chilling time)
Serving Size: 1

Ingredients:
- 1 ripe banana, mashed
- 2 tablespoons chia seeds
- 1/2 cup coconut milk
- 1 tablespoon shredded coconut
- 1 tablespoon chopped mixed nuts
- 1 tablespoon honey or agave syrup

Instructions:
1. In a bowl, mix the mashed banana, chia seeds, coconut milk, shredded coconut, and honey.
2. Stir well to combine all ingredients.

3. Let the mixture sit for 5 minutes, then stir again.

4. Cover and refrigerate for at least 2 hours or overnight.

5. Before serving, top with chopped nuts and an extra sprinkle of shredded coconut.

6. Dive into the tropical flavors of coconut banana nut chia pudding!

CHAPTER TWO

Lunch options to Support Parkinson's Health

Grilled Salmon Salad

Recipe 1:

Grilled Salmon Salad with Mixed Greens

Ingredients:
- 4 (4 oz) salmon filets
- 8 cups mixed greens (spinach, arugula, romaine)
- 1 cup cherry tomatoes, halved
- 1/2 cucumber, sliced
- 2 tbsp crumbled feta cheese
- 2 tbsp sliced almonds

- 2 tbsp balsamic vinaigrette

Nutrition (per serving):
Calories: 320
Total Fat: 18g
Saturated Fat: 4g
Cholesterol: 70mg
Sodium: 420mg
Total Carbs: 12g
Fiber: 4g
Protein: 30g

Cooking Time: 15 minutes
Serves: 4

Instructions:
1. Preheat the grill to medium-high heat.
2. Season salmon filets with salt and pepper.
3. Grill salmon for 4-5 minutes per side, or until cooked through.
4. In a large salad bowl, combine mixed greens, tomatoes, cucumber, feta, and almonds.

5. Top with grilled salmon and drizzle with balsamic vinaigrette.

Recipe 2:

Grilled Salmon Salad with Quinoa and Avocado

Ingredients:
- 4 (4 oz) salmon filets
- 2 cups cooked quinoa
- 1 avocado, diced
- 1 cup cherry tomatoes, halved
- 1/2 red onion, thinly sliced
- 2 cups baby spinach
- 2 tbsp olive oil
- 1 tbsp lemon juice
- Salt and pepper to taste

Nutrition (per serving):
Calories: 390
Total Fat: 22g
Saturated Fat: 4g
Cholesterol: 70mg
Sodium: 320mg

Total Carbs: 25g
Fiber: 6g
Protein: 28g

Cooking Time: 20 minutes
Serves: 4

Instructions:
1. Preheat the grill to medium-high heat.
2. Season salmon filets with salt and pepper.
3. Grill salmon for 4-5 minutes per side, or until cooked through.
4. In a large bowl, combine cooked quinoa, avocado, tomatoes, onion, and spinach.
5. Drizzle with olive oil and lemon juice, and toss to coat.
6. Top salad with grilled salmon.

Recipe 3:

Grilled Salmon Salad with Roasted Vegetables

Ingredients:
- 4 (4 oz) salmon filets
- 2 cups mixed roasted vegetables (bell peppers, zucchini, onions)
- 4 cups mixed greens
- 1/4 cup crumbled feta cheese
- 2 tbsp balsamic glaze
- 1 tbsp olive oil
- Salt and pepper to taste

Nutrition (per serving):
Calories: 350
Total Fat: 19g
Saturated Fat: 5g
Cholesterol: 70mg
Sodium: 480mg
Total Carbs: 16g
Fiber: 5g
Protein: 32g

Cooking Time: 25 minutes
Serves: 4

Instructions:
1. Preheat the grill to medium-high heat.

2. Season salmon filets with salt and pepper.
3. Grill salmon for 4-5 minutes per side, or until cooked through.
4. In a large bowl, combine roasted vegetables and mixed greens.
5. Top with grilled salmon, feta cheese, and drizzle with balsamic glaze and olive oil.

Recipe 4:

Grilled Salmon Salad with Citrus Vinaigrette

Ingredients:
- 4 (4 oz) salmon filets
- 6 cups mixed greens
- 1 orange, segmented
- 1 grapefruit, segmented
- 1/4 cup sliced almonds
- 2 tbsp olive oil
- 2 tbsp orange juice
- 1 tbsp grapefruit juice
- 1 tbsp white wine vinegar

- Salt and pepper to taste

Nutrition (per serving):
Calories: 330
Total Fat: 18g
Saturated Fat: 3g
Cholesterol: 70mg
Sodium: 280mg
Total Carbs: 16g
Fiber: 5g
Protein: 29g

Cooking Time: 20 minutes
Serves: 4

Instructions:
1. Preheat the grill to medium-high heat.
2. Season salmon filets with salt and pepper.
3. Grill salmon for 4-5 minutes per side, or until cooked through.
4. In a large salad bowl, combine mixed greens, orange segments, grapefruit segments, and sliced almonds.

5. In a small bowl, whisk together olive oil, orange juice, grapefruit juice, and white wine vinegar.
6. Drizzle the citrus vinaigrette over the salad and top with grilled salmon.

- Quinoa and Vegetable Stir-Fry

Recipe 1:

Quinoa and Vegetable Stir-Fry with Tofu

Ingredients:
- 1 cup uncooked quinoa
- 1 block (14 oz) extra-firm tofu, cubed
- 2 tbsp olive oil
- 1 red bell pepper, sliced
- 1 cup broccoli florets
- 1 cup sliced mushrooms
- 2 cloves garlic, minced
- 2 tbsp low-sodium soy sauce
- 1 tbsp rice vinegar
- 1 tsp sesame oil

- Salt and pepper to taste

Nutrition (per serving):
Calories: 360
Total Fat: 16g
Saturated Fat: 2g
Cholesterol: 0mg
Sodium: 420mg
Total Carbs: 38g
Fiber: 6g
Protein: 20g

Cooking Time: 30 minutes
Serves: 4

Instructions:
1. Cook quinoa according to package instructions.
2. In a large skillet or wok, heat olive oil over medium-high heat.
3. Add tofu cubes and cook for 3-4 minutes, until lightly browned. Remove tofu from the pan and set aside.
4. Add the bell pepper, broccoli, and mushrooms to the pan. Stir-fry for 5-6

minutes, until vegetables are tender-crisp.

5. Add the garlic and cook for 1 minute, until fragrant.

6. Return the cooked tofu to the pan. Stir in the cooked quinoa, soy sauce, rice vinegar, and sesame oil. Season with salt and pepper.

7. Toss everything together and serve hot.

Recipe 2:

Quinoa and Vegetable Stir-Fry with Chicken

Ingredients:
- 1 cup uncooked quinoa
- 1 lb boneless, skinless chicken breasts, cut into bite-sized pieces
- 2 tbsp vegetable oil
- 2 cups mixed vegetables (broccoli, carrots, snow peas, etc.)
- 2 cloves garlic, minced
- 2 tbsp low-sodium soy sauce

- 1 tbsp honey
- 1 tsp sesame oil
- Salt and pepper to taste

Nutrition (per serving):
Calories: 390
Total Fat: 12g
Saturated Fat: 2g
Cholesterol: 70mg
Sodium: 470mg
Total Carbs: 40g
Fiber: 5g
Protein: 35g

Cooking Time: 25 minutes
Serves: 4

Instructions:
1. Cook quinoa according to package instructions.
2. In a large skillet or wok, heat vegetable oil over medium-high heat.
3. Add the chicken and stir-fry for 5-6 minutes, until cooked through. Remove chicken from the pan and set aside.

4. Add the mixed vegetables to the pan and stir-fry for 3-4 minutes, until tender-crisp.

5. Add the garlic and cook for 1 minute, until fragrant.

6. Return the cooked chicken to the pan. Stir in the cooked quinoa, soy sauce, honey, and sesame oil. Season with salt and pepper.

7. Toss everything together and serve hot.

Recipe 3:

Quinoa and Vegetable Stir-Fry with Shrimp

Ingredients:
- 1 cup uncooked quinoa
- 1 lb peeled and deveined shrimp
- 2 tbsp olive oil
- 2 cups mixed vegetables (bell peppers, zucchini, onions)
- 2 cloves garlic, minced
- 2 tbsp low-sodium soy sauce

- 1 tbsp rice vinegar
- 1 tsp honey
- 1/4 tsp red pepper flakes (optional)
- Salt and pepper to taste

Nutrition (per serving):
Calories: 370
Total Fat: 11g
Saturated Fat: 1.5g
Cholesterol: 190 mg
Sodium: 520mg
Total Carbs: 38g
Fiber: 5g
Protein: 30g

Cooking Time: 25 minutes
Serves: 4

Instructions:
1. Cook quinoa according to package instructions.
2. In a large skillet or wok, heat olive oil over medium-high heat.

3. Add the shrimp and stir-fry for 3-4 minutes, until cooked through. Remove shrimp from the pan and set aside.
4. Add the mixed vegetables to the pan and stir-fry for 4-5 minutes, until tender-crisp.
5. Add the garlic and cook for 1 minute, until fragrant.
6. Return the cooked shrimp to the pan. Stir in the cooked quinoa, soy sauce, rice vinegar, and honey. If using, add the red pepper flakes. Season with salt and pepper.
7. Toss everything together and serve hot.

Recipe 4:

 Quinoa and Vegetable Stir-Fry with Edamame

Ingredients:
- 1 cup uncooked quinoa
- 1 cup frozen shelled edamame
- 2 tbsp sesame oil

- 2 cups mixed vegetables (cabbage, carrots, snow peas)
- 2 cloves garlic, minced
- 2 tbsp low-sodium soy sauce
- 1 tbsp rice vinegar
- 1 tsp grated ginger
- Salt and pepper to taste

Nutrition (per serving):
Calories: 340
Total Fat: 14g
Saturated Fat: 2g
Cholesterol: 0mg
Sodium: 460mg
Total Carbs: 40g
Fiber: 7g
Protein: 15g

Cooking Time: 25 minutes
Serves: 4

Instructions:
1. Cook quinoa according to package instructions.

2. In a large skillet or wok, heat sesame oil over medium-high heat.
3. Add the mixed vegetables and stir-fry for 4-5 minutes, until tender-crisp.
4. Add the garlic and ginger, and cook for 1 minute, until fragrant.
5. Stir in the cooked quinoa, edamame, soy sauce, and rice vinegar. Season with salt and pepper.
6. Toss everything together and serve hot.

 - Chickpea and Roasted Vegetable Bowl

Recipe 1:

 Chickpea and Roasted Vegetable Bowl with Tahini Dressing

Ingredients:
- 1 (15 oz) can chickpeas, drained and rinsed
- 2 cups cubed butternut squash

- 1 red bell pepper, diced
- 1 cup brussels sprouts, halved
- 2 tbsp olive oil
- 1 tsp cumin
- Salt and pepper to taste
- 2 cups mixed greens
- 2 tbsp tahini
- 2 tbsp lemon juice
- 1 tbsp water
- 1 garlic clove, minced
- 1 tbsp maple syrup

Nutrition (per serving):
Calories: 390
Total Fat: 16g
Saturated Fat: 2g
Cholesterol: 0mg
Sodium: 350mg
Total Carbs: 52g
Fiber: 12g
Protein: 14g

Cooking Time: 35 minutes
Serves: 4

Instructions:
1. Preheat the oven to 400°F.
2. Toss the chickpeas, butternut squash, bell pepper, and brussels sprouts with olive oil, cumin, salt, and pepper. Spread on a baking sheet and roast for 25-30 minutes, stirring halfway, until vegetables are tender and lightly browned.
3. In a small bowl, whisk together the tahini, lemon juice, water, garlic, and maple syrup to make the dressing.
4. Divide the mixed greens among 4 bowls. Top each with the roasted vegetables and chickpeas. Drizzle with the tahini dressing.

Recipe 2:

Chickpea and Roasted Vegetable Bowl with Pesto

Ingredients:
- 1 (15 oz) can chickpeas, drained and rinsed

- 2 cups cubed sweet potatoes
- 1 cup cauliflower florets
- 1 cup cherry tomatoes, halved
- 2 tbsp olive oil
- 1 tsp garlic powder
- Salt and pepper to taste
- 2 cups baby spinach
- 1/4 cup basil pesto

Nutrition (per serving):
Calories: 360
Total Fat: 15g
Saturated Fat: 3g
Cholesterol: 0mg
Sodium: 390mg
Total Carbs: 45g
Fiber: 10g
Protein: 13g

Cooking Time: 35 minutes
Serves: 4

Instructions:
1. Preheat the oven to 400°F.

2. Toss the chickpeas, sweet potatoes, cauliflower, and cherry tomatoes with olive oil, garlic powder, salt, and pepper. Spread on a baking sheet and roast for 25-30 minutes, stirring halfway, until vegetables are tender and lightly browned.

3. Divide the baby spinach among 4 bowls. Top each with the roasted vegetables and chickpeas. Drizzle with the basil pesto.

Recipe 3:

Chickpea and Roasted Vegetable Bowl with Avocado Dressing

Ingredients:
- 1 (15 oz) can chickpeas, drained and rinsed
- 2 cups cubed zucchini
- 1 cup sliced mushrooms
- 1 red onion, diced
- 2 tbsp olive oil
- 1 tsp dried oregano

- Salt and pepper to taste
- 2 cups mixed greens
- 1 avocado, mashed
- 2 tbsp lime juice
- 1 tbsp water
- 1 garlic clove, minced
- 1 tsp honey

Nutrition (per serving):
Calories: 380
Total Fat: 18g
Saturated Fat: 2.5g
Cholesterol: 0mg
Sodium: 280mg
Total Carbs: 47g
Fiber: 12g
Protein: 12g

Cooking Time: 35 minutes
Serves: 4

Instructions:
1. Preheat the oven to 400°F.
2. Toss the chickpeas, zucchini, mushrooms, and red onion with olive

oil, oregano, salt, and pepper. Spread on a baking sheet and roast for 25-30 minutes, stirring halfway, until vegetables are tender and lightly browned.

3. In a small bowl, mash the avocado and mix with lime juice, water, garlic, and honey to make the dressing.

4. Divide the mixed greens among 4 bowls. Top each with the roasted vegetables and chickpeas. Drizzle with the avocado dressing.

Recipe 4:

Chickpea and Roasted Vegetable Bowl with Tahini-Lemon Dressing

Ingredients:
- 1 (15 oz) can chickpeas, drained and rinsed
- 2 cups cubed beets
- 1 cup sliced carrots
- 1 cup broccoli florets
- 2 tbsp olive oil

- 1 tsp paprika
- Salt and pepper to taste
- 2 cups arugula
- 2 tbsp tahini
- 2 tbsp lemon juice
- 1 tbsp water
- 1 tsp honey
- 1 garlic clove, minced

Nutrition (per serving):
Calories: 370
Total Fat: 15g
Saturated Fat: 2g
Cholesterol: 0mg
Sodium: 390mg
Total Carbs: 48g
Fiber: 13g
Protein: 13g

Cooking Time: 35 minutes
Serves: 4

Instructions:
1. Preheat the oven to 400°F.

2. Toss the chickpeas, beets, carrots, and broccoli with olive oil, paprika, salt, and pepper. Spread on a baking sheet and roast for 25-30 minutes, stirring halfway, until vegetables are tender and lightly browned.

3. In a small bowl, whisk together the tahini, lemon juice, water, honey, and garlic to make the dressing.

4. Divide the arugula among 4 bowls. Top each with the roasted vegetables and chickpeas. Drizzle with the tahini-lemon dressing.

CHAPTER THREE

Nutritious Dinner Options for Parkinson's Patients

-Baked Chicken with Sweet Potatoes

Recipe 1:

Baked Chicken and Sweet Potato Bites

Ingredients:
- 1 lb boneless, skinless chicken breasts, cut into 1-inch cubes
- 2 medium sweet potatoes, peeled and cut into 1-inch cubes
- 2 tbsp olive oil
- 1 tsp paprika
- 1 tsp garlic powder
- 1/2 tsp dried thyme

- Salt and pepper to taste

Nutrition (per serving):
Calories: 270
Total Fat: 8g
Saturated Fat: 1g
Cholesterol: 65mg
Sodium: 140mg
Total Carbs: 23g
Fiber: 4g
Protein: 27g

Cooking Time: 30 minutes
Serves: 4

Instructions:
1. Preheat the oven to 400°F.
2. In a large bowl, toss the chicken cubes and sweet potato cubes with olive oil, paprika, garlic powder, thyme, salt, and pepper until well coated.
3. Spread the chicken and sweet potato mixture on a baking sheet lined with parchment paper.

4. Bake for 25-30 minutes, stirring halfway, until the chicken is cooked through and the sweet potatoes are tender.
5. Serve hot.

Recipe 2:

 Baked Chicken and Sweet Potato Medley

Ingredients:
- 4 (6 oz) boneless, skinless chicken breasts
- 3 medium sweet potatoes, peeled and cut into 1-inch cubes
- 1 red onion, sliced
- 2 tbsp olive oil
- 1 tsp dried rosemary
- 1 tsp dried thyme
- Salt and pepper to taste

Nutrition (per serving):
Calories: 350
Total Fat: 10g

Saturated Fat: 1.5g
Cholesterol: 90mg
Sodium: 190 mg
Total Carbs: 30g
Fiber: 5g
Protein: 35g

Cooking Time: 40 minutes
Serves: 4

Instructions:
1. Preheat the oven to 400°F.
2. Place the chicken breasts, sweet potato cubes, and red onion slices in a large baking dish. Drizzle with olive oil and sprinkle with rosemary, thyme, salt, and pepper. Toss to coat.
3. Bake for 35-40 minutes, or until the chicken is cooked through and the sweet potatoes are tender.
4. Serve hot.

Recipe 3:

Baked Chicken and Sweet Potato Stuffed Peppers

Ingredients:
- 4 (6 oz) boneless, skinless chicken breasts, cooked and shredded
- 2 cups cubed sweet potatoes
- 1 cup cooked quinoa
- 1/2 cup diced onion
- 2 cloves garlic, minced
- 1 tsp chili powder
- 1/2 tsp cumin
- Salt and pepper to taste
- 4 bell peppers, halved and seeded

Nutrition (per serving):
Calories: 330
Total Fat: 7g
Saturated Fat: 1g
Cholesterol: 70mg
Sodium: 200mg
Total Carbs: 36g
Fiber: 6g
Protein: 32g

Cooking Time: 50 minutes
Serves: 4

Instructions:
1. Preheat the oven to 375°F.
2. In a large bowl, combine the shredded chicken, cubed sweet potatoes, cooked quinoa, onion, garlic, chili powder, cumin, salt, and pepper.
3. Stuff the mixture into the halved bell peppers and place them in a baking dish.
4. Bake for 40-45 minutes, or until the peppers are tender and the filling is heated through.
5. Serve hot.

Recipe 4:

Baked Chicken and Sweet Potato Skewers

Ingredients:
- 1 lb boneless, skinless chicken thighs, cut into 1-inch cubes

- 2 medium sweet potatoes, peeled and
cut into 1-inch cubes
- 1 red onion, cut into 1-inch pieces
- 2 tbsp olive oil
- 1 tsp smoked paprika
- 1/2 tsp ground cumin
- Salt and pepper to taste

Nutrition (per serving):
Calories: 290
Total Fat: 10g
Saturated Fat: 2g
Cholesterol: 85mg
Sodium: 180mg
Total Carbs: 21g
Fiber: 3g
Protein: 29g

Cooking Time: 25 minutes
Serves: 4

Instructions:
1. Preheat the oven to 400°F.

2. Thread the chicken cubes, sweet potato cubes, and onion pieces onto skewers.
3. In a small bowl, mix together the olive oil, smoked paprika, cumin, salt, and pepper.
4. Brush the skewers with the spiced oil mixture.
5. Arrange the skewers on a baking sheet lined with parchment paper.
6. Bake for 20-25 minutes, turning occasionally, until the chicken is cooked through and the vegetables are tender.
7. Serve hot.

- Lentil Soup with Kale

Recipe 1:

Classic Lentil and Kale Soup

Ingredients:
- 1 cup dry brown lentils, rinsed

- 4 cups low-sodium vegetable or chicken broth
- 1 tbsp olive oil
- 1 onion, diced
- 2 carrots, peeled and diced
- 2 celery stalks, diced
- 3 garlic cloves, minced
- 1 tsp ground cumin
- 1 tsp dried thyme
- 1/4 tsp red pepper flakes (optional)
- 4 cups chopped kale, stems removed
- Salt and pepper to taste

Nutrition (per serving):
Calories: 270
Total Fat: 5g
Saturated Fat: 1g
Cholesterol: 0mg
Sodium: 350mg
Total Carbs: 40g
Fiber: 12g
Protein: 16g

Cooking Time: 45 minutes
Serves: 4

Instructions:

1. In a large pot, combine the lentils and broth. Bring to a boil, then reduce heat and simmer for 15-20 minutes, until lentils are tender.

2. In a separate skillet, heat the olive oil over medium heat. Add the onion, carrots, celery, and garlic. Cook for 5-7 minutes, until vegetables are softened.

3. Add the sautéed vegetables, cumin, thyme, and red pepper flakes (if using) to the pot with the lentils. Simmer for 10 more minutes.

4. Stir in the chopped kale and cook for 5 more minutes, until the kale is wilted.

5. Season with salt and pepper to taste.

6. Serve hot.

Recipe 2:

Lentil and Kale Soup with Sausage

Ingredients:
- 1 cup dry green lentils, rinsed

- 4 cups low-sodium chicken broth
- 1 tbsp olive oil
- 1 lb Italian sausage, casings removed
- 1 onion, diced
- 3 garlic cloves, minced
- 2 tsp dried oregano
- 1 tsp dried basil
- 4 cups chopped kale, stems removed
- Salt and pepper to taste

Nutrition (per serving):
Calories: 360
Total Fat: 15g
Saturated Fat: 4g
Cholesterol: 45mg
Sodium: 630mg
Total Carbs: 33g
Fiber: 11g
Protein: 25g

Cooking Time: 45 minutes
Serves: 4

Instructions:

1. In a large pot, combine the lentils and chicken broth. Bring to a boil, then reduce heat and simmer for 15-20 minutes, until lentils are tender.
2. In a separate skillet, heat the olive oil over medium heat. Add the Italian sausage and cook, breaking it up with a spoon, until browned, about 5-7 minutes.
3. Add the onion and garlic to the sausage and cook for 2-3 minutes, until fragrant.
4. Transfer the sausage mixture to the pot with the cooked lentils. Stir in the oregano and basil.
5. Add the chopped kale and cook for 5 more minutes, until the kale is wilted.
6. Season with salt and pepper to taste.
7. Serve hot.

Recipe 3:

Lentil and Kale Soup with Sweet Potatoes

Ingredients:
- 1 cup dry red lentils, rinsed
- 4 cups low-sodium vegetable broth
- 1 tbsp olive oil
- 1 onion, diced
- 2 sweet potatoes, peeled and cubed
- 3 garlic cloves, minced
- 1 tsp ground cumin
- 1 tsp smoked paprika
- 4 cups chopped kale, stems removed
- Salt and pepper to taste

Nutrition (per serving):
Calories: 320
Total Fat: 6g
Saturated Fat: 1g
Cholesterol: 0mg
Sodium: 380mg
Total Carbs: 52g
Fiber: 11g
Protein: 15g

Cooking Time: 40 minutes
Serves: 4

Instructions:

1. In a large pot, combine the lentils and vegetable broth. Bring to a boil, then reduce heat and simmer for 10-15 minutes, until lentils are tender.

2. In a separate skillet, heat the olive oil over medium heat. Add the onion and sweet potato cubes. Cook for 5-7 minutes, until the vegetables are softened.

3. Add the garlic, cumin, and smoked paprika to the skillet. Cook for 1 minute, until fragrant.

4. Transfer the sautéed vegetables to the pot with the cooked lentils. Stir to combine.

5. Add the chopped kale and cook for 5 more minutes, until the kale is wilted.

6. Season with salt and pepper to taste.

7. Serve hot.

Recipe 4:

Lentil and Kale Soup with Quinoa

Ingredients:
- 1 cup dry brown lentils, rinsed
- 1 cup dry quinoa, rinsed
- 4 cups low-sodium vegetable broth
- 1 tbsp olive oil
- 1 onion, diced
- 3 garlic cloves, minced
- 2 tsp ground ginger
- 1 tsp ground coriander
- 4 cups chopped kale, stems removed
- Salt and pepper to taste

Nutrition (per serving):
Calories: 350
Total Fat: 8g
Saturated Fat: 1g
Cholesterol: 0mg
Sodium: 300mg
Total Carbs: 50g
Fiber: 13g
Protein: 19g

Cooking Time: 40 minutes
Serves: 4

Instructions:

1. In a large pot, combine the lentils, quinoa, and vegetable broth. Bring to a boil, then reduce heat and simmer for 15-20 minutes, until the lentils and quinoa are tender.

2. In a separate skillet, heat the olive oil over medium heat. Add the onion and cook for 3-4 minutes, until softened.

3. Add the garlic, ginger, and coriander to the skillet. Cook for 1 minute, until fragrant.

4. Transfer the sautéed onion mixture to the pot with the cooked lentils and quinoa. Stir to combine.

5. Add the chopped kale and cook for 5 more minutes, until the kale is wilted.

6. Season with salt and pepper to taste.

7. Serve hot.

- Baked Cod with Roasted Vegetables

Recipe 1:

Baked Cod with Roasted Vegetables

Ingredients:
- 4 (6 oz) cod filets
- 2 cups cubed sweet potatoes
- 1 cup Brussels sprouts, halved
- 1 red bell pepper, sliced
- 1 red onion, sliced
- 2 tbsp olive oil
- 1 tsp dried thyme
- 1 tsp paprika
- Salt and pepper to taste
- Lemon wedges for serving

Nutrition (per serving):
Calories: 320
Total Fat: 9g
Saturated Fat: 1.5g
Cholesterol: 80mg
Sodium: 290 mg
Total Carbs: 28g
Fiber: 6g
Protein: 32g

Cooking Time: 35 minutes
Serves: 4

Instructions:
1. Preheat the oven to 400°F.
2. In a large baking dish, toss the sweet potatoes, Brussels sprouts, bell pepper, and onion with olive oil, thyme, paprika, salt, and pepper.
3. Roast the vegetables for 20 minutes, stirring halfway.
4. Push the vegetables to the sides of the baking dish and place the cod filets in the middle.
5. Bake for an additional 12-15 minutes, until the cod is opaque and flakes easily with a fork.
6. Serve the baked cod with the roasted vegetables and lemon wedges.

Recipe 2:

Baked Cod with Lemon-Garlic Roasted Vegetables

Ingredients:
- 4 (6 oz) cod filets
- 2 cups cubed zucchini
- 1 cup cherry tomatoes, halved
- 1 cup sliced mushrooms
- 3 garlic cloves, minced
- 2 tbsp olive oil
- 1 tbsp lemon juice
- 1 tsp dried oregano
- Salt and pepper to taste

Nutrition (per serving):
Calories: 280
Total Fat: 10g
Saturated Fat: 1.5g
Cholesterol: 80mg
Sodium: 290 mg
Total Carbs: 15g
Fiber: 4g
Protein: 35g

Cooking Time: 30 minutes
Serves: 4

Instructions:

1. Preheat the oven to 400°F.

2. In a large baking dish, combine the zucchini, cherry tomatoes, mushrooms, and garlic. Drizzle with olive oil, lemon juice, oregano, salt, and pepper. Toss to coat.

3. Roast the vegetables for 15 minutes.

4. Push the vegetables to the sides of the baking dish and place the cod filets in the middle.

5. Bake for an additional 12-15 minutes, until the cod is opaque and flakes easily with a fork.

6. Serve the baked cod with the lemon-garlic roasted vegetables.

Recipe 3:

Baked Cod with Rosemary Roasted Vegetables

Ingredients:
- 4 (6 oz) cod filets
- 2 cups cubed butternut squash
- 1 cup broccoli florets

- 1 red onion, sliced
- 2 tbsp olive oil
- 2 tsp chopped fresh rosemary
- 1 tsp garlic powder
- Salt and pepper to taste

Nutrition (per serving):
Calories: 300
Total Fat: 8g
Saturated Fat: 1g
Cholesterol: 80mg
Sodium: 280mg
Total Carbs: 22g
Fiber: 5g
Protein: 35g

Cooking Time: 40 minutes
Serves: 4

Instructions:
1. Preheat the oven to 400°F.
2. In a large baking dish, toss the butternut squash, broccoli, and red onion with olive oil, rosemary, garlic powder, salt, and pepper.

3. Roast the vegetables for 25 minutes, stirring halfway.
4. Push the vegetables to the sides of the baking dish and place the cod filets in the middle.
5. Bake for an additional 12-15 minutes, until the cod is opaque and flakes easily with a fork.
6. Serve the baked cod with the rosemary roasted vegetables.

Recipe 4:

 Baked Cod with Mediterranean Roasted Vegetables

Ingredients:
- 4 (6 oz) cod filets
- 2 cups cubed eggplant
- 1 cup halved cherry tomatoes
- 1 cup sliced zucchini
- 1/2 cup kalamata olives, sliced
- 2 tbsp olive oil
- 1 tsp dried oregano
- 1 tsp dried basil

- 2 cloves garlic, minced
- Salt and pepper to taste

Nutrition (per serving):
Calories: 310
Total Fat: 12g
Saturated Fat: 2g
Cholesterol: 80mg
Sodium: 420mg
Total Carbs: 18g
Fiber: 6g
Protein: 35g

Cooking Time: 35 minutes
Serves: 4

Instructions:
1. Preheat the oven to 400°F.
2. In a large baking dish, combine the eggplant, cherry tomatoes, zucchini, and olives. Drizzle with olive oil and sprinkle with oregano, basil, garlic, salt, and pepper. Toss to coat.
3. Roast the vegetables for 20 minutes, stirring halfway.

4. Push the vegetables to the sides of the baking dish and place the cod filets in the middle.

5. Bake for an additional 12-15 minutes, until the cod is opaque and flakes easily with a fork.

6. Serve the baked cod with the Mediterranean roasted vegetables.

-Stuffed Bell Peppers with Ground Turkey

Recipe 1:

Classic Stuffed Bell Peppers

Ingredients:
- 6 medium bell peppers (mix of colors)
- 1 lb ground turkey
- 1 cup cooked rice
- 1 small onion, diced
- 2 cloves garlic, minced
- 1 (15 oz) can diced tomatoes

- 1 tsp dried oregano
- 1 tsp dried basil
- Salt and pepper to taste
- 1 cup shredded cheese (cheddar or mozzarella)

Nutritional Information (per serving):
- Calories: 280
- Total Fat: 10g
- Saturated Fat: 4g
- Cholesterol: 75mg
- Sodium: 480mg
- Total Carbs: 25g
- Fiber: 5g
- Protein: 25g

Cooking Time: 60 minutes
Serving Size: 1 stuffed pepper

Instructions:
1. Preheat the oven to 375°F.
2. Cut the tops off the bell peppers and remove the seeds and membranes. Place the peppers in a baking dish.

3. In a skillet, cook the ground turkey over medium heat until browned. Drain any excess fat.
4. Add the cooked rice, onion, garlic, diced tomatoes, oregano, basil, salt, and pepper. Mix well.
5. Stuff the mixture into the hollowed-out bell peppers.
6. Top the peppers with shredded cheese.
7. Bake for 30-40 minutes, or until the peppers are tender and the cheese is melted and bubbly.

Recipe 2: Tex-Mex Stuffed Bell Peppers

Ingredients:
- 6 medium bell peppers (mix of colors)
- 1 lb ground turkey
- 1 cup cooked brown rice
- 1 (15 oz) can black beans, drained and rinsed
- 1 cup salsa
- 1 tsp chili powder
- 1 tsp cumin

- Salt and pepper to taste
- 1 cup shredded cheddar cheese

Nutritional Information (per serving):
- Calories: 300
- Total Fat: 12g
- Saturated Fat: 5g
- Cholesterol: 70mg
- Sodium: 590mg
- Total Carbs: 30g
- Fiber: 7g
- Protein: 26g

Cooking Time: 55 minutes
Serving Size: 1 stuffed pepper

Instructions:
1. Preheat the oven to 375°F.
2. Cut the tops off the bell peppers and remove the seeds and membranes. Place the peppers in a baking dish.
3. In a skillet, cook the ground turkey over medium heat until browned. Drain any excess fat.

4. Add the cooked rice, black beans, salsa, chili powder, cumin, salt, and pepper. Mix well.
5. Stuff the mixture into the hollowed-out bell peppers.
6. Top the peppers with shredded cheddar cheese.
7. Bake for 25-30 minutes, or until the peppers are tender and the cheese is melted and bubbly.

Recipe 3:

Mediterranean Stuffed Bell Peppers

Ingredients:
- 6 medium bell peppers (mix of colors)
- 1 lb ground turkey
- 1 cup cooked quinoa
- 1 (15 oz) can diced tomatoes
- 1/2 cup crumbled feta cheese
- 1/4 cup chopped fresh parsley
- 2 cloves garlic, minced
- 1 tsp dried oregano
- Salt and pepper to taste

Nutritional Information (per serving):
- Calories: 260
- Total Fat: 11g
- Saturated Fat: 3g
- Cholesterol: 75mg
- Sodium: 520mg
- Total Carbs: 20g
- Fiber: 4g
- Protein: 24g

Cooking Time: 50 minutes
Serving Size: 1 stuffed pepper

Instructions:
1. Preheat the oven to 375°F.
2. Cut the tops off the bell peppers and remove the seeds and membranes. Place the peppers in a baking dish.
3. In a skillet, cook the ground turkey over medium heat until browned. Drain any excess fat.
4. Add the cooked quinoa, diced tomatoes, feta cheese, parsley, garlic, oregano, salt, and pepper. Mix well.

5. Stuff the mixture into the hollowed-out bell peppers.
6. Bake for 25-30 minutes, or until the peppers are tender.

Recipe 4:

Italian Stuffed Bell Peppers

Ingredients:
- 6 medium bell peppers (mix of colors)
- 1 lb ground turkey
- 1 cup cooked brown rice
- 1 (15 oz) can diced tomatoes
- 1/2 cup grated Parmesan cheese
- 2 cloves garlic, minced
- 1 tsp dried basil
- 1 tsp dried oregano
- Salt and pepper to taste

Nutritional Information (per serving):
- Calories: 270
- Total Fat: 9g
- Saturated Fat: 3g
- Cholesterol: 80mg

- Sodium: 560mg
- Total Carbs: 24g
- Fiber: 5g
- Protein: 25g

Cooking Time: 55 minutes
Serving Size: 1 stuffed pepper

Instructions:
1. Preheat the oven to 375°F.
2. Cut the tops off the bell peppers and remove the seeds and membranes. Place the peppers in a baking dish.
3. In a skillet, cook the ground turkey over medium heat until browned. Drain any excess fat.
4. Add the cooked rice, diced tomatoes, Parmesan cheese, garlic, basil, oregano, salt, and pepper. Mix well.
5. Stuff the mixture into the hollowed-out bell peppers.
6. Bake for 25-30 minutes, or until the peppers are tender and the filling is hot.

CONCLUSION

The complexity and multifaceted nature of Parkinson's disease have long posed significant challenges for researchers and clinicians alike. However, the recent advancements in our understanding of this debilitating condition offer a glimmer of hope for a brighter future. By unmasking the intricate web of genetic, environmental, and neurological factors contributing to Parkinson's, we have laid the groundwork for more targeted and effective interventions.

The identification of key genetic mutations and the exploration of environmental triggers have shed light on the underlying mechanisms driving the development and progression of Parkinson's disease. This knowledge has opened up new avenues for early detection, personalized treatment approaches, and preventive strategies. The refinement of diagnostic tools, such as advanced neuroimaging techniques and biomarker analysis, has enabled earlier and more accurate diagnoses, allowing for timely interventions that can potentially slow the disease's course.

Furthermore, the advancements in neuroprotective therapies, including novel pharmacological agents and innovative neuromodulation approaches, hold the promise of preserving and even restoring neuronal function in individuals with Parkinson's. The exploration of stem cell-based therapies and regenerative medicine techniques offers the tantalizing prospect of reversing the neurodegenerative processes, potentially restoring lost motor and cognitive abilities.

Alongside these medical breakthroughs, the pivotal role of multidisciplinary care teams and the empowerment of patients and their families cannot be overstated. The integration of comprehensive, patient-centered approaches that address the physical, emotional, and social needs of individuals with Parkinson's disease has been instrumental in improving quality of life and enhancing overall well-being.

As we continue to unravel the complexities of Parkinson's disease, the future holds immense promise. With sustained research efforts, collaborative partnerships, and a steadfast commitment to improving the lives of those affected, we are poised to make significant strides in conquering this debilitating condition. The road ahead may be long and arduous, but with each incremental advance, we inch closer to a world where Parkinson's disease is not just managed, but ultimately conquered, restoring hope and dignity to those who bravely face this challenge.